You're Fat!
Now Lose It!

You're Fat! Now Lose It!

✦

Help! I'm Fat! Now I Need To Lose It

70 pounds in 6 Months—GONE

M. J. Specogna

iUniverse, Inc.

New York Lincoln Shanghai

You're Fat! Now Lose It!
Help! I'm Fat! Now I Need To Lose It

iUniverse books may be ordered through booksellers or by contacting:

iUniverse
2021 Pine Lake Road, Suite 100
Lincoln, NE 68512
www.iuniverse.com
1-800-Authors (1-800-288-4677)

Because of the dynamic nature of the Internet, any Web addresses or links contained in this book may have changed since publication and may no longer be valid.

You should not undertake any diet/exercise regimen recommended in this book before consulting your personal physician. Neither the author nor the publisher shall be responsible or liable for any loss or damage allegedly arising as a consequence of your use or application of any information or suggestions contained in this book.

ISBN: 978-0-595-47231-4 (pbk)
ISBN: 978-0-595-91514-9 (ebk)

Printed in the United States of America

Thanks to Schindler for being an enthusiastic and willing walk partner, and for making the bit go fast.

"If your friends and family get fat, chances are you will too"

—Alicia Chang, Researcher 2007.

Contents

Preface

I want to share my secret with you on losing weight. I want to help you win the battle. Following this program will help you shed pounds just as I did. Need evidence, look at my before and after pictures. Good luck to you.

A startling study in mid 2007, while writing this book, revealed that obesity is contagious. That is right. The study by Alicia Chang, funded by the U.S. National Institute on Aging, and published in the New England Journal of Medicine was summarized as follows: "If your friends and family get fat, chances are you will too, researchers report in a startling new study that suggests obesity is "socially contagious" and can spread easily from person to person".

The chances of you becoming obese rise to 57 percent if your friend is obese, 40 percent if your sibling becomes overweight and 37 percent if your spouse becomes obese.

The study suggests that obesity in North America, where two thirds of the population falls within the obese category, is not genetic based but rather socially based.

You're fat now it's time to lose it will help you lose weight. If you lose it, most likely those around you will also, if the study is correct.

Let us start on a better road to health. The study pointed out that obesity claims 300,000 lives a year, second only to smoking. The study suggests, as pointed out in later chapters, food is an addiction similar to smoking.

Intro

I was fat and did not realize it. Or, perhaps I did know I was overweight but I refused to accept this fact. I felt that I needed to lose some weight, but was in denial that I was actually obese. I also kept procrastinating about losing weight and becoming a healthier person.

I am not a doctor. I am not a fitness guru. I am not a colonics specialist. I am an average person like you. I lost 70 pounds in 6 months. You can too!

Important: you must be an adult to follow this program. Children that are still growing cannot follow this program. Do Not Follow This Program if you are under 21.

A number of personal reasons motivated me to start a diet. My reasons may have been much different from what your reason(s) are to lose weight today. Both of our motivating reasons could be the same, it does not matter. What matters is that you have taken a step, a first step in your journey to becoming a healthier person, by committing to losing some weight.

WHY CHOOSE THIS BOOK?

There are many self-help books, videos, seminars, diets, and diet books in the market place on losing weight and becoming a healthier person. There are so many choices to pick from in making your commitment a reality. All these choices make the whole process of becoming a healthier person and losing weight confusing.

You may have tried a number of other diets or programs. Regardless of whether they have worked or not, you are looking for another choice or you would not be reading this book.

This program worked for me. If I did it, you can too! It works, it is hard but stay motivated, and it will work. There is no magic overnight success. However, if you stay true to this program, you will lose weight.

THIS BOOK WILL HELP YOU LOSE WEIGHT

This book will help you lose weight. This book will help you lose weight with a simple diet program and a very simple fitness program. There are no colonics involved, no cleansing programs involved, no high cost programs, or unreasonable requirements to follow this program. There are no outrageous fitness requirements. No bodybuilding program is included, and no running for hours on end.

This book will help you lose weight.

I accumulated a lot of extra weight over the years. I have tried to explain the steps to losing the extra weight that you have accumulated over the years using the program that helped me. This book outlines simple steps in a weight loss program. However, even though the program is simple it is at the same time a very difficult endeavor. The whole process is mentally hard since you have to alter your eating habits slightly. The alteration of eating habits is not drastic just a slight variation in the types of food eaten. You can't be eating the chocolate bars, the potato chips, or the one-pound hamburgers.

The motivation for this book is to give you a real opportunity to lose weight, which will lead you to feeling healthier. The program is not complicated. You will not need to undertake a demanding physical exercise program, just a realistic simple, timesaving, general movement program worked into your busy day.

WHAT DO YOU GET?

You get to lose weight inexpensively. You get to keep extra money in your pocket by not purchasing as much food as you have in the past. You become a healthier person. You do not need to become a fitness guru to follow this program. You do not need to cleanse for this program. You do not need to do colonics or enemas for this program. You lose weight by following this program. You become healthier by following this program.

WHAT DO I OFFER YOU?

So, you are asking yourself what do I offer you that no one else does. In a way, that is what I asked myself before I even attempted to write this short self-help book. The reasons I gave myself for writing this book perhaps answers this question. I was motivated to lose the weight I gained from snacking, overeating, and unhealthy food eating. My health deteriorated from being overweight. I want to share the steps of my weight loss with you, hopefully to inspire you to follow the simple program to weight loss and feeling healthier.

I want to share with you how I lost the weight. You can do it if I did. Look at my before and after pictures. You should be able to notice a big difference in my appearance, and weight levels! Alter your eating habits as I did. Alter your eating habits and follow the program as outlined and you will lose weight. You will notice a significant change in your appearance and health.

I recall nutrition and life eating lessons taught to me by my parents, and nutritionists. However, with so many food choices, and great cuisine I threw all the good eating habits out of my mind over time. Once I made the realization that I needed to lose weight, I researched basic information to ensure a healthy program. I will reveal the program later in the book, as well as the basic information gleaned from so many sources researched. You do not need to spend as much time and money, as I did researching, since I give you all you need to know in simple terms.

First Step—You're fat, now start the program.

The first step is to understand that you have a weight problem. Most likely you are obese as I was.

You need to accept you are obese. Call it overweight, but the fact is you are on an unhealthy course that will ruin your health and wallet, and could possibly lead to your premature death! Whether you fall in the obese or overweight category, it is time to start your journey to losing weight. Your acceptance of being overweight or obese is essential to staying committed to this program.

THIS PROGRAM WILL WORK FOR ANYONE!

This program will work for anyone. If I did it, you can!

I was very inactive and had self-imposed limited mobility for one year before I started my program. I was not motivated to be active. I was unhealthy, as I could not walk down the street without heavy breathing and labored walking. My legs would hurt, or throb after a short 2-minute walk. Even during those moments, I would be in denial about my obesity.

I became a healthier and lighter person from following my program. I spent a lot of time researching the best methods of weight lose and found the best one that is tried and true, and just tweaked it to fit my lifestyle. My lifestyle is typical of the average person, so it will fit you well.

This program works. I lost 70 pounds in 6 months. You simply have to look at the before and after headshots of myself to acknowledge this fact. I followed this program, became a healthier person, and successfully lost weight. If I can do it, anyone can!

70 pounds in 6 Months—GONE

Losing 70 pounds in 6 months may not seem like a major feat since all self-help programs do have people featured that have the same or better results. I have a before picture, where I actually added a further 15 pounds before I started my program, and an after picture which you have seen all over this book.

You can see from my face and the fit of my clothes how much heavier I was than I currently am. I started my journey at 265 pounds. At 5'8", that is the obese level. I was overweight. I was in denial. At the time, I did not believe I was overweight. It took time for me to realize that the troubled breathing caused by simple walking was due to my weight. I realized I needed to do something or I may not be around to see my children grow older.

I also used to snore, but since I lost my weight, I do not snore anymore. Could it be the extra weight I had was causing me to snore when sleeping on my back? I do not know I am not an expert, but it seems bizarre that after losing the weight I do not snore anymore. Perhaps you will find that you also do not snore after losing weight. How great would that be?

HARD JOURNEY, BUT IF I DID IT, SO CAN YOU!

I used the word journey earlier because any weight loss program is difficult, with many ups and downs experienced. The first thing you need to understand and I do not say this shocking statement to be mean, only to have you realize the truth. You're fat and it's time to lose it!

Do not be offended. I found I had to tell myself this statement and believe it, before I could commit fully to losing weight and embark on the journey of losing weight.

You have to tell yourself the following statement repeatedly. I am fat and it is time to lose it! If you feel bad, feel hurt or are upset about this statement that is great. The truth hurts. Time for you to accept the fact you are overweight. If not, stop reading right now, and do not start again until you have admitted you are obese and you want to do something about it.

The journey will see you have self-doubts along the way. Or you will believe that you are not losing weight. And, on the odd occasion, you will believe that no results are visible. But, during any of these self-doubts, you have to shake those thoughts and stay committed. You will be surprised with the results of perseverance.

Accept YOU Are Overweight—You Want To Embark On The Hard Journey

Congratulations!

You have accepted the fact you are overweight. Now you need to embark on the journey. The hard work of following this great weight loss program where you may not notice results right away, but after a few weeks those around you will notice some results.

Re-iterating, following the program is hard. You will be tempted to feed your desire for the great tasting cuisine, snacks, and unhealthy food that are around us everywhere. You will have to stay focused to the program. Breaking old habits is hard. But understand that all the hard work will payoff with your own after picture! You will feel healthier, and look great.

You will have to alter your lifestyle and your eating habits. You will need to make a slight change in your lifestyle by including a simple fitness program. You will need to make an extreme change in your eating habits. It really is not easy to stay focused on this program. You have to maintain discipline, and stay focused. If you maintain the program and stay disciplined, you will attain a healthy weight level, feel healthy, and have a super after picture to show off.

How Do I Know You Will Lose Weight?

I know you will lose weight because I did. I lost weight the same way you will. All you have to do is follow the program and understand these facts:

You need to alter your eating habits

You need to alter you lifestyle a bit

You have to stay focused

You have to follow the program

You have to remember the program

It is easy to lose focus. Just look around you and you will see others who are battling the same focus problem. These people, as we did, forgot the basic principles of eating food. We all lost focus, and discipline, and did not realize that we were, or are, in fact obese.

It is easy to give up. It is also easy to lose the pounds if you follow the program and remember your goal(s). Follow the program and you will lose weight. It is as simple as that. Stay focused on your goals and stick with the program.

Easy To Give Up and Be In Denial

You may look at yourself in the mirror as I had in the past, and not see an obese person. It is so easy not to criticize ourselves, but the labored movements, and clothes size do not lie. The obese weight levels tabulated are realistic values so scoffing at the values is being in denial.

If I can lose 70 pounds in 6 months, and 6 inches off my waistline, you can lose the same or more. I am not any different than you are. I just focused on my goal, and developed a diet program after research, that works and anyone can follow. I do not lead an active lifestyle, as my work is sedate. I am typical of the average North American person.

THE HEAVIER YOU ARE—THE MORE YOU LOSE FASTER

The best part about this program is the fact that the heavier you are the faster you will lose the weight! This is only true if you follow the program. You have to admit this is a great benefit. The more you weigh the more weight you lose faster.

SET YOUR GOAL

It is important to have a generic goal. You should outline your goal as follows. My goal is to lose some weight.

Or, I would like to become a healthier person.

Or, I want to look at a before picture taken today and in 3 months I want to take an after picture and see results of my weight loss program.

Or, I want to have my clothes fit me properly.

Or, I need to lose weight to take pressure off my vital organs, so I stay alive longer and enjoy life.

All those listed generic goals are realistic goals.

Setting a goal with a number of pounds lost in a number of months is not a realistic goal.

Those number types of goals are not realistic since following the program could cause you some difficulties. You are altering your lifestyle slightly and altering your eating habits in a major way to follow the program, so these two factors could cause you difficulties.

With this in mind, there will be some days where you may waver slightly from your program. The waver may be a necessity. It is a calling, from your body, not to overdo the program but feed the body's need. The important fact to remember is a waver is a good thing and that you are just replenishing your body some additional nutrients. Doing this will help you to remain focused.

Generic goals help you stay focused. Goals with numbers are not realistic.

It is time to list your goals. Write out your goal or goals below. Remember set realistic generic goals, not using numbers of pounds to lose by a certain number of days. List your goals. Think about them seriously. You will need to look at your goals often to help stay focused.

Some examples of my own personal goals were:

My written were the following:

To follow the program.

Not be tempted with overeating, snacking, or eating foods that are bad for me.

To commit to stay focused until I have lost enough weight so as I am not on the obese side of the chart, and so that I feel healthy while simply walking.

To have my clothes fit me without my belly hanging over my belt line.

Those were my generic basic goals. In fact, in regards to the last goal, all my clothes ended up being seven sizes to big after my program.

Time to write out your goals, and remember keep them generic. In addition, list any other goals you may have that will result from losing a large amount of weight. Write them below so that you can reread them later to stay focused. For example, you may want to be able to walk with your kids. Maybe you want to prove to others you can be focused? Write the goals here:

WAVERING OFF THE PROGRAM SOMETIMES IS OK

I mentioned earlier that you might waver off the program. Some days your body will be calling out to you to waver from the program. What I mean by this statement is the fact that your body will need energy to maintain the program. Some days that energy requirement may be much more than the program is providing. You will need to eat a few more calories than you usually would, to quell your body hunger pains. In your own mind, you will probably be able to address the situations that arise at that moment in time. Deal with the hunger pain. That is ok. Feel free to waver sometimes. Eat proper low calorie high volume food, no manufactured products.

You will know when your body is calling for extra energy so you should feed it based on this diet program. Remember feed the body low calorie high volume food only, even when you waver. No manufactured foods. Feeling guilty about wavering is good, just stay focused and remember your goal or goals, reread them often.

No Overnight Changes Will Happen—Get That Straight

You will notice results slowly. Perhaps, in the first 30 days there maybe no noticeable results, but you have to understand the program is slowly having an affect on your body, and on how you look. One source of information, during my research, suggested that the first fat lost is internal fat around vital organs. This fat needs to be lost before weight is lost on the exterior. In regards to the amount of fat stored around our organs, everyone is different.

To prove the program is working weigh yourself. You will amaze yourself that even though it is not noticeable, you have in fact lost weight. You know the program is working. Just remain focused.

I found once I had lost 25 pounds that my health improved dramatically. For me that was 3 weeks into my program. However, when I looked in the mirror I did not see any changes. The reason I did not notice any changes was that I was still obese. It was hard for me to see a change in my body since I was 70 pounds overweight and had only lost 25 pounds. I did feel at that time that my health definitely improved as my breathing difficulty disappeared.

Remember this fact. A weight scale does not lie. If you are lighter in weight when you weigh yourself, you are winning.

When Will You Notice Results?

When will you notice results? That will be different for everyone, and depends on the program you choose. Nevertheless, remember the weight scale does not lie so you will know you have lost weight.

Just because you believe you look no different in the mirror does not mean you have not lost weight. Stay focused you are on the right path. If your scale tells you that you are 10 pounds lighter, but you look the same, in your mind, in the mirror, you know the scale is right.

What do you need?

First, you will need to be committed to your goal or goals. You have to stay positive. You need to commit. You need to remember your goal or goals as you outlined earlier. Go and reread them now. You need to remember them everyday. You need to read the goals everyday, and stay committed. It is hard, but if you want some encouragement look at my before and after pictures. You too will have before and after pictures, and you will amaze yourself but you have to follow the program, stay focused.

You will need a weight scale so you can weigh yourself. You will need to change your eating habits. You will need to change your lifestyle a little bit. Change is such a harsh word, alter is probably a better word. You will need to alter your eating habits and alter your lifestyle a little bit. Your eating habits refers to the elimination of snack times, snack foods, high energy low substance foods, and almost all fast food.

WEIGHT SCALES

Digital weight scales are great, but any scale is ok. There are always some discrepancies in scales so make sure you use the same scale when you weigh yourself. Different scales have different calibrations so you cannot compare one scale weight number to another.

The best scales are mechanical eye-level weight scales. The type found in a doctor's office. These scales maintain the calibration, or if lose the calibration due to air pressure it can be calibrated manually. The weight reading will be accurate at all times and will be the same on any calibrated mechanical eye-level weight scale.

Just remember. You may have a fluctuation in weight numbers some days. These fluctuations are ok. The fluctuations are simply how the body works. As long as you maintain the program and stay focused, you will win and notice great results. Remain focused on your program. You may not be able to notice any results but your body is changing slowly if you are following the program.

If your weight numbers are higher after awhile, and consistently stay at higher levels than when you started, unless you have initiated a weight lifting program and are adding muscle, then you obviously are not following the program or are cheating with snacks or between meal eating. This would definitely suggest that you have wavered off your program too much, or are not following the program at all.

You may also find you are losing too much weight too rapidly so you will need to alter your program to keep from losing too much weight too fast. I know sounds like an ideal situation but you can develop serious health problems if losing weight too fast.

You will also need to replace some of the drinks you consume daily with water. You still can keep a limited amount of carbonated or sugary drinks in your daily diet. However, the majority of your liquids must be water, or a mix added to water, like "Tang". You can add any low calorie mix to water to add flavor. Realize that man has lived solely with water as a beverage since the beginning of time, so water could be a full daily replacement to the manufactured sugary drinks we all love.

Recommended daily water intake for a person is eight glasses, so it is good to drink as close to eight glasses of water a day as possible. In addition, water has zero calories, so the more you drink the fewer calories you have consumed!

The Program—The only way

This program revolves around monitoring calories and some minor exercise. You also have to alter the types of food and quantity of food consumed on a daily basis to get great results. A simple fitness program will speed up the burning of calories. The simple fitness program consists of walking.

After a lot of research, there is no other way to lose weight or burn fat other than monitoring calories. Roughly counting the number of calories you consume, and the rough number you burn, on a daily basis will return a new and healthy you.

Calories are definitely the only way to losing weight without committing to a vigorous workout regiment. None of us can start a hard workout program. We are either overweight or obese. Any significant exercise regiment is out of the question. We have become sedentary over the years and any significant exercise program will stress our organs and body.

Since we have been sedentary, and not trained our bodies in any physical activity, we could have any number of injuries occur if we suddenly start a vigorous physical fitness program. As a matter of fact the first few days or week, we may only be able to complete our simple fitness program of walking, for only five minutes. That is ok, since that is how I started, and look at the results, 70 pounds gone in 6 months.

Like you, I did not have enough time in the day to commit to a vigorous army type workout anyways. Not that any of you, or I, could start those hard-core cardio workouts yet. You have been inactive for too long. You cannot suddenly put stress on bone and muscle that is required by any vigorous workouts. But, after a few months on the program you could start one of those types of fitness regiments if you so desire.

For the moment, for the start of this calorie-counting program and the fitness portion of the program, you can do realistic minor exercise anytime of the day. The program tells you how little exercise to do to lose weight. The exercise is simple. Just walk!

Walking is all that is required of you. Follow the diet program and the fitness program consisting of simple walking, and you will get results like those that I did. Simple walking plus following the calorie-counting program and you will have results like mine or better. Remember I lost 70 pounds in 6 months.

MULTI-VITAMIN TO ENSURE HEALTHY

You will also need a good multi-vitamin to keep on hand in case you need to supplement your diet. If you do not take in 1,500 calories a day, you will need a multi-vitamin a day to stay healthy. The 1,500 calories a day is the minimum caloric intake per day a person must consume to maintain a healthy body. Many Doctors and Organizations World wide have reported this number. So if you go below that number take a multi-vitamin.

The multi-vitamin will help include any minerals lacking in your diet.

THE PROGRAM STARTS NOW

The calorie counting method of weight loss is a phenomenal program. Many books disclose the calorie-counting method, and many diet programs utilize the calorie-counting method but do not necessarily disclose this fact. I know calorie-counting works; it helped me become a healthy person and helped me lose 70 pounds in 6 months. The facts listed below, we know from numerous reliable medical associations, and scientific associations all garnered from scientific data and work for decades.

It is fact that our bodies need calories to live.

It is also a fact that the body uses calories 24 hours a day.

It is also fact that unused Calories are stored as fat.

It is fact that all food has calories except for water, which has zero calories.

Medical professionals established all these basic calorie facts previously. But nowhere except in this book, is the calorie counting method described in easy to learn terms. No other book describes the calorie-counting method in as much detail as is outlined in this book. You need to accept those four facts listed above.

NO MAGIC

No magic pill will let you eat as much as you want and burn calories for you as you lead a sedated lifestyle. Controlling your caloric intake and some minor walking everyday will work visible wonders fast.

Remember that no magic pill will destroy the calories consumed. No magic pill will reduce our fat without our reduction of calories in our diet. It is better to consume food with low calories and large volumes, not small volume foods with high calories, because we need to feel full so as not to consume more bad calories.

ACCEPT THE FACTS

You have to accept all those facts outlined above. Commit to no more foods that are high calorie and small volume in size. More foods with higher volume and fewer calories are ideal.

Like you, I never accepted those facts and I became obese. I believed the doctors who said only eat certain foods high in protein to lose weight. Eating foods that are higher in protein do not help you lose weight. These other diets never worked for me, and I know they do not work for you.

I never wanted to educate myself on simple calorie counting. Calorie counting is so simple because the government requires all foods sold to contain the calories per serving size. The serving sizes are stated by measuring cup size, so it is easy to figure out the amount of food to cook to get the desired calories. So counting your calories is simple. You cannot keep blinkers on and not count your calories. The information is there so use it.

When I did decide to educate myself on calorie counting, after I accepted the facts listed above. I could not find any book, literature, or information of any kind that outlined in simple terms how the calorie-counting program works. I have outlined in the most simplest of terms the information that took me months to find, and I have added it all in this book. The calorie counting method works, look at my before and after pictures.

I used it and I lost 70 pounds in 6 months!

Calorie counting is the backbone of your program. You will need to count calories. This does not mean you have to use a small scale to measure out portions of food. Rough estimates work well as long as they are realistic estimates. Everyone has measuring cups, so put it to use.

EASY TO REMEMBER

The way to lose weight is to use energy. Use energy and you burn calories. The more calories you burn in a day than you eat, will burn the fat you have stored. Your body stores all the calories you do not burn in one day. The calories are stored as fat. The fat stored on our bodies is unburned calories we have eaten.

To burn fat, and to lose weight you need to burn more calories per day than you consume. Remember that if you consume less than 1,500 calories a day you will need to add a multi-vitamin to your program.

Counting calories sounds simple and many nutritionists, doctors, and medical associations recommend this method of weight loss. Many books outline calorie counting, but do not give you any realistic advice, nor is there ever any proof it has worked for someone. You see my before and after pictures so you know it works, and that is without any major fitness program, The results were obtained by solely following the program of calorie counting and walking.

Many books on the market also recommend the calorie counting method of weight loss, but do not disclose that fact. The method of weight lose is hidden in simply providing you a meal program to follow.

Many books recommend a high level of exercise to lose weight. The level of exercise promoted by these other books, are so unrealistic for the average person. This causes people like us to stop with the whole diet process, or delay a weight loss program for a while. How can anyone who has not done any sort of exercise for years, or who is obese start doing a one-hour program? The fitness programs in other books are far too complicated, unrealistic and ridiculously physically hard, that people stop the whole diet program. How many of you have experienced that with other programs? With the calorie-counting program, you will not quit it because of the fitness program.

This calorie-counting program is simple and easy to follow. It can be hard to follow though if you lose focus. It becomes hard because you are counting calories and consuming far less food than you have in the past. You also have to stop snacks and in between meal eating.

It can be hard to follow this program, stay focused. Stay focused on your goals. Focus on counting the calories. Focus on how many calories you eat in a day. Focus on how many calories you burn in a day. These facts will help you lose weight. These facts helped me lose 70 pounds in 6 months.

Burn more calories in one day than you consume and you will lose weight. This is the calorie-counting program described in one sentence.

If your body burns more calories than are consumed in a daily basis, you will lose weight. You will win the battle. Easier said than done, but I will explain how to do it.

Each pound of fat your body has stored equals 3,500 calories. Every pound of fat is only 3,500 extra calories that were not consumed in energy by your body. If you consume 6,000 calories today and only burn 1,000 calories, you have added over one and a half pounds of fat to your body today. Those 5,000 calories are very hard to burn, it is easier to add calories so remember count your calories.

There are numerous free calorie counters on the net. The online calorie counters help to understand the number of calories each food item contains, and the number of calories burned in any exercise including our simple walking exercise. Jogging does not burn any more calories than walking so that fact should have you giggling if you see people jogging while you walk.

HOW DO I BURN CALORIES?

Every daily activity burns calories. Remember this fact, that every activity, from sleeping to sitting to walking to sex, all burns some calories. All daily activities burn calories. However, the number of calories burned is not large. So stay disciplined. Eating a few chocolate bars, a bag of chips and consuming a few pop add pounds to our body. Eating these products puts more high calorie, low volume, foods into our system. These high calories make it harder to burn the calories off to attain weight loss. Plus the high calorie foods have smaller volume and do not fill us up.

It is easier to eat calories than it is to burn the calories. This is a fact, just look at your obese self.

THE HEAVIER YOU ARE—THE FASTER YOU LOSE WEIGHT

This is such a wonderful fact. The heavier you weight the faster you will lose weight. The reason is that the heavier you are, the more your body has to work. The more your body has to work the more calories you burn. The more calories you burn, the more weight you lose. Only if you limit the number of calories you consume.

Remember that each pound you weigh is 3,500 calories. The heavier you are means you burn 3,500 calories faster. Therefore, if you weigh over 500 pounds you will burn 3,500 calories faster than a person who weights 250 pounds. Only true if you limit the number of calories you consume, and the total number of calories burned in one day, is more than the total number of calories consumed in one day.

JUST SITTING, SLEEPING AND WALKING BURNS CALORIES!

Sleeping and sitting burns some calories, and the heavier you are, the more calories you will burn! Walking burns just as much calories as a slow jog so why start any program jogging? Exactly, it does not make sense to start with jogging when you can just as easily walk and burn the same calories.

Look at just the simple act of sleeping. The following data came from the US Medical Association.

Realize that if you are 265 pounds sleeping for 5 hours burns roughly 550 calories. However, if you weigh 190 pounds, sleeping for 5 hours will burn only 399 calories. If you sleep ten hours, multiply by two. If you weigh 500 pounds and sleep 10 hours, you burn 2,100 calories. Remember to check an online calorie counter website to determine your calorie consumptions based on your height and weight, and level of activities.

From these figures, you can see your body burns calories even when you sleep. Your weight will affect how much calories you burn for each activity, and the less you weigh the less calories you burn. The less you weigh, the fewer calories you burn, means the fewer calories you can consume.

As you progress in the program from a high weight to a lower weight, you will realize the amount of calories burned in a day will also be less than the amount burned when you weighed more. Therefore, you will need to alter your calorie consumption.

Back to the activity of sleeping, the lighter you become means that sleeping will burn less of your daily calorie intake so you have to adjust by doing more walking or less calorie consumption.

Further examples of how much calories you burn from sleeping. If you weigh 425 pounds, you lose 945 calories sleeping for 5 hours. If you weigh 600 pounds, you burn 1,470 calories sleeping for 5 hours. Both these two weights burn more calories in ten hours of sleeping than most people over 60 consume in one day!

So does this mean you sleep all day? No. I simply point out the fact that your body requires calories just to stay alive and burns calories every second of the day in any activity. However, the number of calories burned for any activity is very small compared to the amount of calories in most food.

Many free websites offer calculating the calories burnt for an activity based on your weight and the length of an activity. This can be a great planning guide. Since the web addresses change so much, it is easier for you to use a search engine to find one that works for you.

Sleeping burns calories and so does sitting. If you weigh 250 pounds and sit for 16 hours in a day, you will burn 1,600 calories.

In one day, just sleeping and sitting will see you burn approximately 2,000 calories, if you weigh 250 pounds. However, realize if you eat the wrong foods, you could consume those 2,000 calories from some bad food choices in one meal.

At least we all burn calories everyday just maintaining an existence, or working. We all need to become healthier and lose weight or we would not be looking for an answer to our problem. Use the food packaging that outlines the calories per serving. Use an online calculator for foods that do not have a consumer guide label.

Meats are high in calories so use the calculators to know what calorie amount you are consuming. Use the calorie counters to know the amount of calories burned for any activity. Remember to lose weight you need to burn more calories than consumed and to lose weight you need to lose 3,500 calories extra than consumed to lose a pound.

YOUR FITNESS PROGRAM

Your program will require calorie counting. You need to keep track of calories you eat. You need to know the size of a serving printed on the side of a package and the number of calories in the serving size. You need to remember the rough amount of calories burned every day from simple everyday tasks. Everyday tasks like sleeping, sitting, and walking, all use energy so these activities all burn calories.

Walking consumes calories, and the heavier you are, the more calories you will burn. The more calories you burn the more weight you will lose. If you use the guide of 100 calories per 20 minutes of walking, you can determine the number of calories burned in one hour of walking. This will help you outline a goal of minutes per day of walking to burn calories per day. Walking is not as simple as it sounds if you are overweight.

Walking can be a challenge if you are obese. Start walking to burn calories and get blood circulating. Walk only for a few minutes at a time to start. You will feel sore after if you are obese so do not overdo walking at the beginning. Over days, as you walk for more minutes, you will still be sore. Eventually you will walk for a certain amount of minutes and not feel sore. Just because you can walk for five minutes and not feel sore does not mean you can walk ten minutes without feeling sore. Walk moderately for the first few days then build it up. You are working out your obese body using calories so your body becomes sore. The more time you spend walking and feel sore the MORE calories you are burning. The MORE calories you are burning the MORE WEIGHT YOU ARE LOSING!

Walking will be difficult to start. Stay focused. Your body may become sore the more minutes you walk. This soreness could make you believe walking is hard. Stay Focused. Keep walking but cut back the minutes so you are not so sore. Over a few days, you will be able to move to longer timed walks.

You do not have to walk a marathon and you do not have to walk outside. Walking around your apartment or house is good enough. Standing instead of sitting will burn a few more calories a day, plus will help your legs get stronger to walk for longer periods.

Using the rough, 100 calories burned for every 20 minutes of walking, will help you determine how many calories you are burning. If you commit just to walk around your apartment or, office, or your block, for cumulative one hour or two hours in one day you will consume 400 to 800 calories.

The more you walk the more calories you will burn. The heavier you are the more you will burn in the same time as I have given the 100 calories per 20 minutes for a 200-pound person. The calories burned increase if you weigh more. Again this rough estimate is for a person around 200 pounds so the heavier you are the more calories you will burn.

WALKING—IS YOUR FITNESS PROGRAM

That is the most strenuous exercise you will have to do while on this calorie-counting program. It does not have to be fast walking. Trust me; just starting a walking program will be difficult for you. So please start a program with minimal walking for the first while. I would say just do maximum 5 minutes at any one time to start if you are over 500 pounds. Maybe 5 minutes of non-stop walking is too much. Do minimal walking for a few short minutes to start and work your way up to five minutes non-stop walking. From there try adding extra minutes. A person weighing over 200 pounds could start with a 15-minute non-stop walking session.

Again, walking around your bedroom or apartment is good enough. After awhile you can head outside to walk and walk for more minutes. Walking is important in this program as it helps to either burn the fat accumulated over time or burn the calories consumed in one day. Do not forget, walking and all other activities including sleeping and sitting burn calories. Walking burns more calories over a shorter time period, and puts less stress on obese body frames than jogging or running. Do not be fooled, it is hard work walking for extended periods if you have not done any type of physical work or fitness for a while and harder if you are obese.

The reason you start with a low number of minutes walking is the fact your body will be sore from walking. It sounds silly you may say, that from a "simple 5 minute walking session how can my body feel sore". If you have not moved around for years that short five minutes will be huge, trust me you will feel sore. So do not over do the walking immediately, work up the time spent walking over a few weeks. If your body feels ok, then increase it each day, it is up to you. Do not stop walking.

You also need to know that one pound of fat is roughly 3,500 calories. To be winning everyday, you need to ensure the number of calories you eat and burn equals a negative number. So you need to burn more calories per day. And, if you burn more than 3,500 calories than you have consumed, you will burn 1 pound of fat.

Number of calories burned, from all activities in one day, LESS the number of calories consumed in one day, has to equal 3,500 calories or more in one day to lose 1 pound of weight.

Realize that the heavier you are the more calories you will burn from sleeping, sitting, and walking. You can and will have to, control the amount of calories you consume to lose weight. It is hard to stay focused because your body will be calling out to you to consume more calories but you will have to remain focused on your goal(s).

You will have to remember the goals that you wrote down earlier, reread them everyday. The wanting is like an addiction, and it can be very hard to overcome the desire to eat. Eating is an addiction; and can be a strong urge.

The study by Alicia Chang, mentioned in the foreword, points out the possibility that obesity is a social disease and possibly an addiction.

A good way to avoid the desire to eat is to stop buying manufactured food products that can fit in the palm of your hand but contain 3 times the calories that two handfuls of rice or pasta would
contain. Which of the two sizes of food do you think make our
body feel full? You had better know that two handfuls would make
you feel fuller than one handful! All high calorie low volume foods
are to be avoided on you calorie-counting diet. Only eat low calorie,
large volume food.

Palm Sized Meat or Manufactured Food=Same Calories as 6 or 2 handfuls of Rice or Pasta!

Meat also is very high in calories. Meat that fits in the palm of your hand will have the same number of calories as 6 handfuls of rice or pasta! Different types of meat exist, pork, beef, chicken, turkey, and wild game. The different meats have different levels of calories, pork is the highest calorie food, and turkey is the lowest, per serving size. Fish is a separate food and has benefits and negatives. Fish should replace a meat product some days, but documented high mercury levels in fish means eat fish sparingly. Tuna however is a high protein fish, and high calorie food, so if you are not weight lifting to gain muscle, avoid it.

An important fact to understand is that an 8-ounce steak, the size of a hand, contains over 600 calories. Pork chops that are 8 ounces in weight have 1,400 calories. Any meat is high in calories. Meat should be limited because of the amount of calories each meat product contains. The fewer calories you eat, the less weight you will add to your body, the easier to burn more calories than are consumed in one day!

You can keep meat in your diet but on a limited basis. The portions have to be smaller than the palm of you hand. That size of portion is more than the recommended daily allowance for a person by Medical Associations worldwide. Since you have eaten more than that amount of meat for years, you do not need meat for a few weeks, or months!

Pasta, oatmeal, and white rice, pre-cooked, have around 200 calories per cup. Pre-cooked means in its hard-uncooked self. Uncooked product expands to a few times that size. The amount of this food you get to eat will fill you up faster. Think about it. 200 calories of rice, pasta, or oatmeal fill your body up. These are low calorie high volume foods we need to eat on our calorie-counting diet.

The cup of carbohydrates producing these calories will be far greater in volume that high calorie meat products thus alleviating your hunger. Sauces, without meat or fish, also have minimal calories so you can add as much as you want for taste and still be less than 100 calories per spread of sauce. Same with mustard, ketchup, mayonnaise, and salad dressings.

You can eat the pasta and rice, with added vegetables, tomato sauce, or white sauce, as these calories can be negligible. There are so many rice's from all over the world, and they give different textures and flavours, just do the calorie reading homework. Stay away from manufactured rice products, which are high in calories. The point is, carbohydrates fill your hunger with low calories and good energy. Meat products fill your body with huge numbers of calories but will not satisfy underlying hunger since it is such a small quantity and will not give you the full feeling. You will still feel hunger because you are not full.

LET TRI-ATHLETES AND ATHLETES EAT MANUFACTURED FOOD PRODUCTS

You are not a tri-athlete or an athlete so why are you eating manufactured food products like granola bars, fruit roll-ups, and mixed cold cereals?

The most tri-athleting you have done is pulling your clothes on, washing yourself up, and eating. So stop eating granola bars, energy bars, or chocolate bars. These bars all mean huge calories leaving you with that hungry feeling. Huge calories mean a big, fat, obese tri-athlete.

A granola bar that has 400 calories will only make you burp and still leave you hungry. We all know that. Eating a chocolate bar means we ate some more calories we will never burn, or have a harder time burning. Sure, they taste great. The reason they taste great is because the companies making them put flavors in there that they know you will like. The better it tastes the more they sell, and they want repeat business. The problem is, the companies and people running them do not care about our health or worry how many calories we eat. If they did, why would these products have the same amount of calories as part of a sit-down meal and yet still leave us feeling hungry? As reported food may be addictive, so be careful what you eat.

Manufactured food products include chips, snacks, granola bars, also many frozen dinner packages. All these manufactured foods, are un-natural. All un-natural products have huge calories because they are man made products. Huge calories for a small portion of food that just makes it harder for you to lose the weight is a very bizarre concept sold to us consumers. In fact, the more of those manufactured products you eat, the fatter you get. We do not need these products in any diet or as a food source, so drop them from your calorie consumption, meals.

Another bonus for cutting manufactured foods from your diet is the fact you put money back in your wallet, meaning more savings. If you do not like saving money you can send me some money for helping you lose weight.

The best way to stop eating and craving manufactured foods is by not purchasing them. If you do not have them around the house, you will not be able to eat them. If you cannot eat them, you will not add the ridiculous amount of calories in those items.

Stop buying those products and you will be amazed at how much money you save. If you are happy with the results of following my program in this book, send me some of that money with a before and after picture. It will be the best money you ever saved, and you will have some money to show your new self to the world! Trust me; you will need a new wardrobe if you follow the program properly.

WATER HAS **NO** CALORIES

Water has no calories. This is an incredible fact. We can drink water and we are not consuming any calories. Our bodies need water and it has no calories, this is wonderful. If water is too bland for you, then add a mix. Be careful with the mixes also, because again many can be loaded with huge calories and a lot of sugars and salts. Do some homework on a mix.

It is much better to drink water than manufactured drinks that have calories. You do not have to eliminate all the manufactured drinks, but replace some with water, and keep track of the calories these drinks have. That way you know how many calories a day you are consuming by eating and drinking.

This makes knowing how much calories you need to burn to lose weight easier. It is great to go through the day minding your calories but not good to then suddenly consume five cans of pop, each with 120 calories per can. That consumption defeats the purpose.

To clarify this point better. If you consume only 2,000 total food calories in one day but then drink 5 cans of pop, you have added a full 600 to 1000 calories to your total daily calorie intake. That means you will consumed up to 3,000 calories in one day. Therefore, it is better to avoid too many servings of the manufactured drinks in your daily diet.

Remember in 20 minutes of walking you only burn 100 calories. To burn the five cans of pop calories you would need to walk for 2 to 5 hours non-stop. It is hard enough walking for 20 minutes non-stop. I know that right now you cannot stop laughing. Try walking for 20 minutes non-stop first, before you assume you can do it. You have to promise if you try, you will walk non-stop for at least a full five minutes. When you are done, drink a glass of water, and relax. No eating, just relax. Stop thinking it is easy to burn the calories. It is difficult to burn the calories. It is hard so stay focused.

Stay Focused

The program consists of counting calories. It is good enough to estimate the amount of calories consumed by reading the packaging on foods. It is important to remember 3,500 calories equal one pound. It is important to remember that for every 20 minutes of walking you burn only 100 calories.

Finally, a minimum of calories you must consume by eating or drinking in one day is at least 1,500 calories and if not, you need to take a multi-vitamin. You must also not go less than 1,000 calories of proper food intake per day. Remember also, that water contains no calories. No individual under 21 should follow these calorie numbers of 1,500 per day, because children and teens all need a wide range of food and calorie intake. Following these guidelines could be dangerous. Not recommended.

These are the basic facts of calorie counting. To lose weight you need to consume (eat) less calories than you burn.

Typical day Menu Program

A typical day for a 250-pound person on this program could be the following.

A ½ cup of oatmeal for breakfast equals roughly 200 calories. Coffee and a juice another 150 calories, net calories consumed for breakfast is 350.

Walk for 20 minutes in morning equals 100 calories burned, a daily net of 250 calories consumed so far today.

Lunch, one cup of rice, with vegetables, or one cup of pasta, both equal 300 calories, and a manufactured drink 150 calories, net for the day 700 calories, total calories eaten so far in the day is 800.

Walk for 20 minutes results in 100 calories burned making the net daily calories consumed only 600.

Dinner, a portion of meat or chicken, 800 calories, with 1 cup or rice, pasta or potatoes, 200 calories, a manufactured drink 150 calories, equals a total of 1,150 calories for the meal, 1,950 calories consumed all day, but a net total calories of only 1,750 for the day.

Walking for an additional 20 minutes will burn a further 100 calories, meaning a net intake of 1,650 calories for the day.

Sleeping for 8 hours will consume 800 calories. For the 24-hour period, your net consumption of calories is 850 calories. Any sort of work, even just sitting for the remainder of the day would see a majority of those calories burned. You still will not have lost any weight today because you have to burn more than 3,500 calories to lose one pound of fat.

From this eating program, you will not burn any weight unless you either reduce calorie consumption by cutting back the higher calorie food, manufactured drink, or, increase the amount of time you walk. Remember, you can walk back and forth in your office or around your house to burn the calories. The walking burns calories in a ratio of 100 calories per 20 minutes. Therefore, the more minutes you walk in a day, the more calories you will burn. You will also burn calories from your daily work, and movement. So it is quite possible, that even with this meal and fitness program, you will burn weight over a few days and even more so over a few weeks.

Recall that just sitting burns calories. If you just sit for the remainder of the day at an office job, you could burn up to 3,000 calories. From simple sitting for 8 hours and this menu program, you will certainly lose 1 pound a day, if you work in a high-paced environment. The more movement you do, the more weight you will lose faster. And, the heavier you are the more weight you lose faster.

Note also that the less high calorie food, like meat you eat, and drink of manufactured drinks, the more calories you will burn in one day.

If you weigh over 500 pounds, the program above will actually result in you only having a net 100 calories consumed in 24 hours since from your body weight your body burns more calories in one day than a 250-pound person. Calories burned from sitting, or an office job, would be twice as much as a 250-pound person.

If we include the calories burned from sitting at an office job for 8 hours, you could burn up to 6,000 calories, or close to 2 pounds of fat! Any movement, above simple sitting or office work tasks, you do in a day, will increase the calories burned.

If you remove, the size of the meat portion in the menu you will be losing weight faster since 800 calories disappears from your consumption. If you walk for more minutes at anytime during the day, or overall in the day, you will also reduce more weight each day since you are burning more calories. If you remove the manufactured drinks from your diet and stick to 8 glasses of water a day you will lose even more weight. It is simple math by counting calories.

In the above menu program, the total consumed daily calories are at least 1,950 calories. This is far above the minimum 1,500 calories per day consumed as recommended by doctors and medical associations worldwide. To eliminate more calories, you would cut back on the meat serving, or even cut it out of your diet for a few days. Eliminate the manufactured drinks and you will reduce calorie intake and burn weight easier since you are not drinking as many calories everyday.

It is hard work to reduce weight. After 20 minutes of walking, you have only burnt 100 calories. Remember how hard it is to burn 100 calories and you will stay focused on the amount of calories you consume. This will help you remain focused on the program.

TO BURN WEIGHT MEAL PROGRAM

To burn weight in one day for a 250-pound person, follow this program.

Breakfast: ½ cup of oatmeal, or dry cereal or 1 medium sized pancake with syrup, two pieces of toast with jam or peanut butter. These all equal 200 to 300 calories and should leave you feeling full. Drink some water, rather than coffee, milk, or juice, for a few days.

Drink 8 glasses of water per day. If water is too bland for you, then add a mix, but study them carefully.

Walk for 20 minutes, or after a few days up to 1 hour, this will result in 100 to 300 calories burnt.

Lunch, have 1 cup rice or pasta with any type of sauce, a sandwich with one slice of meat, preferably chicken and one thin slice of cheese, this would equate to 300 to 400 calories.

Walk for 20 minutes to 1 hour, this will increase the calories burnt by an additional 100 to 300 calories.

Dinner, 1 cup rice or pasta or handful of potatoes, or two hands of French fries, with palm sized chicken or meat, add veggies to rice, or side of veggies, this will be from 800 to 1,200 calories of consumption.

Walk for 20 minutes to 1 hour to burn 100 to 300 calories.

Sleep for 8 hours, this will burn 800 calories. Total calories consumed today were 1,500 to 1,900 calories. Total burnt calories were 1,100 to 1,700 calories. Net calories are 200 to 400 calories. Again, any sedentary work, sitting will burn an additional up to 3,000 calories in one day.

Repeat the same menu everyday; alter the meals between these products, Oatmeal, simple dry cereal, pancakes, french toast, rice (white, brown, any kind), pasta (only durum without additives, no manufactured additional items), potatoes (mashed, roasted, any cooking method), and french fries. Cut back to eating a meat product only once every few days. Meats are very high in calories, so eat them sparingly.

Increase the amount of walking to a few hours a day. Again, you can walk in your apartment or house while watching TV. If you walk for a total of 4 or 5 hours in one day, just walking, you will burn 1,500 calories. If you keep the meat in your diet, and sleep for the 8 hours, you will be negative 200 to 400 calories a day. This does not include calories burned in other activities during the day that you would normally do, such as just sitting, which we know burns as much as 3,000 calories in one day.

This meal program would result in you losing 1 pound of weight a day.

If you eliminate the meat, you will be negative 1,000 to 1,200 calories in one day. With these calories burned and your sitting calories of up to 3,000 calories burned per day, you will lose 6 pounds in 5 days.

To increase weight loss faster, you can scale back the amount of calories eaten in a day by arranging the size of each portion during the three meals. You can skip breakfast or a lunch every few days, but take the multi-vitamin if you fall below 1,500 calories per day.

The weight loss will become more apparent over time. Each day of greater calorie burn off rather than calorie consumption, and depending on your daily physical work, or movement, those calories burned will increase your weight loss.

For the first few weeks, stay true to the program. Later you can indulge with a burger once in awhile. After a few months, you can move to eating some more meat products, but still count the calories. After a few months, you will have worked up to walking faster, and for longer intervals, and possibly doing some jogging or running. These increased levels of movement will burn more calories and stimulate the food consumed to add some muscle replacing the fat burned.

BURN WEIGHT MEAL PROGRAM FOR ANYONE WEIGHING 500 POUNDS OR MORE

You can follow the same meal program as the 250-pound person. You may initially just walk for 5 minutes non-stop. Any walking, throughout the day, for non-stop periods, even around your office cubicle, is good physical activity to help lose weight while following the calorie-counting program.

Since you weigh much more, the 20 minutes of walking will actually burn a bit more than 100 calories, so the more you walk after a few weeks the faster you will burn calories and lose weight. If you sit for 8 hours, you will be burning up to 6,000 calories. If you have any other movement other than sitting, the calories burned will increase.

Following the meal program for the 250 person, you will be consuming 1,500 to 1,900 calories.

In 8 hours, you will burn 1,600 calories sleeping. Walking, the 3 times of 20 minutes will burn another 300 calories. The sitting for 8 hours will burn up to 6,000 calories. Your total burnt calories for the day will be 7,900 calories.

The eaten calories of 1,500 to 1,900 and the burnt calories of 7,900, equals a total loss of 6,000 to 6,500 calories per day. You will lose almost 2 pounds a day!

In 3 days, you will lose 6 pounds. In 30 days, you will lose 60 pounds. If you skip a few meals over the next few weeks and cut out meat, you will lose more weight. Over a few months you will find burning calories and weight will be slower since you weigh less.

This is a long journey and you can see from my before and after pictures that anybody can do it. Just remain focused. It is easy to eat and add calories but it is hard to burn the calories and lose the weight. Remember the hard work to burn calories, make it just as hard to let yourself eat unnecessary foods, or between meals. That will help you be successful in your weight loss program.

Remember how easy it is to eat high calorie foods, and how hard it is to burn the calories. Good luck in your diet program, please let me know how it went, or how you are doing.

978-0-595-47231-4
0-595-47231-1